MW01534342

ER Nurses

by Julie Murray

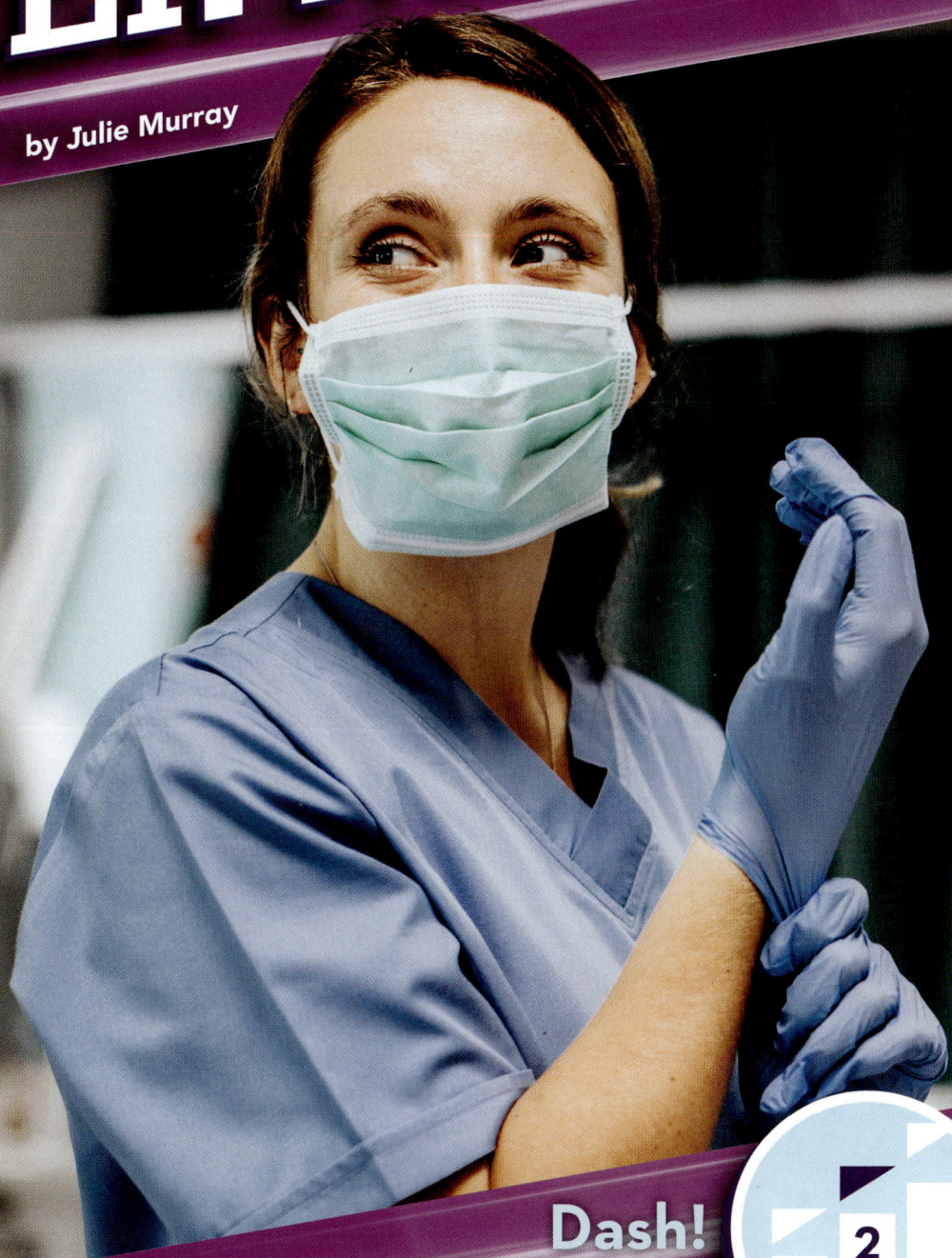

Dash!
LEVELED READERS
An Imprint of Abdo Zoom • abdobooks.com

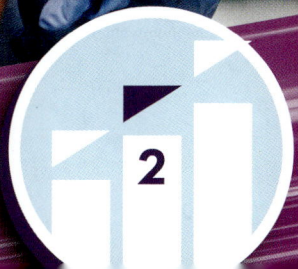

2

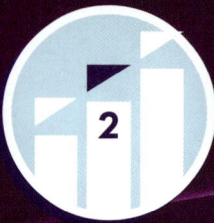

2 Dash!
LEVELED READERS

Level 1 – Beginning
Short and simple sentences with familiar words or patterns for children who are beginning to understand how letters and sounds go together.

Level 2 – Emerging
Longer words and sentences with more complex language patterns for readers who are practicing common words and letter sounds.

Level 3 – Transitional
More developed language and vocabulary for readers who are becoming more independent.

THIS BOOK CONTAINS RECYCLED MATERIALS

abdobooks.com

Published by Abdo Zoom, a division of ABDO, PO Box 398166, Minneapolis, Minnesota 55439.
Copyright © 2021 by Abdo Consulting Group, Inc. International copyrights reserved in all countries.
No part of this book may be reproduced in any form without written permission from the publisher.
Dash!™ is a trademark and logo of Abdo Zoom.

Printed in the United States of America, North Mankato, Minnesota.
102020
012021

Photo Credits: iStock, Shutterstock
Production Contributors: Kenny Abdo, Jennie Forsberg, Grace Hansen, John Hansen
Design Contributors: Dorothy Toth, Neil Klinepier, Laura Graphenteen

Library of Congress Control Number: 2020910907

Publisher's Cataloging in Publication Data

Names: Murray, Julie, author.
Title: ER nurses / by Julie Murray
Description: Minneapolis, Minnesota : Abdo Zoom, 2021 | Series: Emergency jobs | Includes online
    resources and index.
Identifiers: ISBN 9781098223052 (lib. bdg.) | ISBN 9781098223755 (ebook) | ISBN 9781098224103
    (Read-to-Me ebook)
Subjects: LCSH: Nurses--Juvenile literature. | Emergency nursing--Juvenile literature. | Emergency medical
    services--Juvenile literature. | Hospitals--Emergency services--Juvenile literature. | Assistance in
    emergencies--Juvenile literature.
Classification: DDC 363.3481--dc23

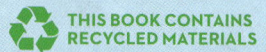

Table of Contents

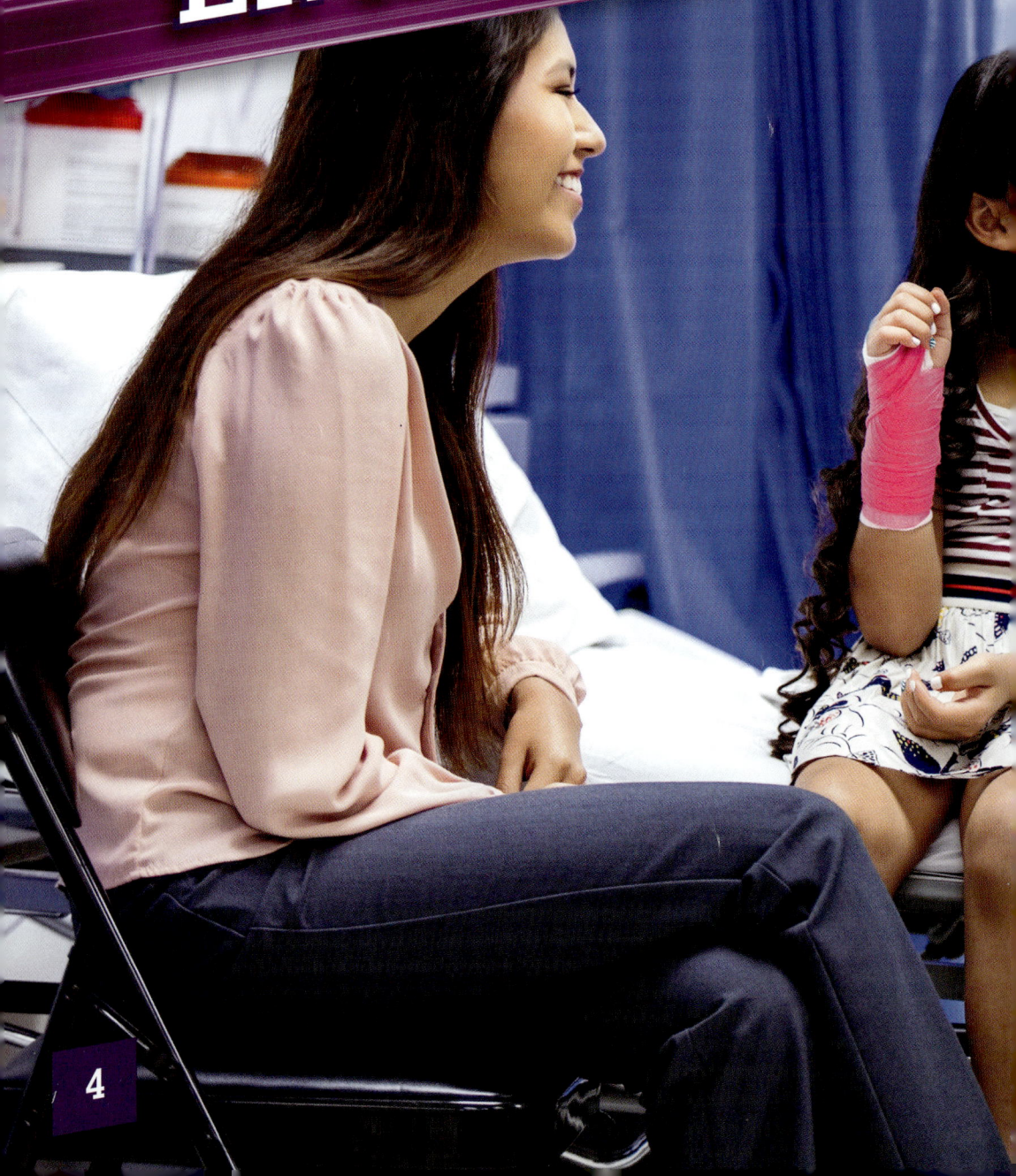

ER Nurses

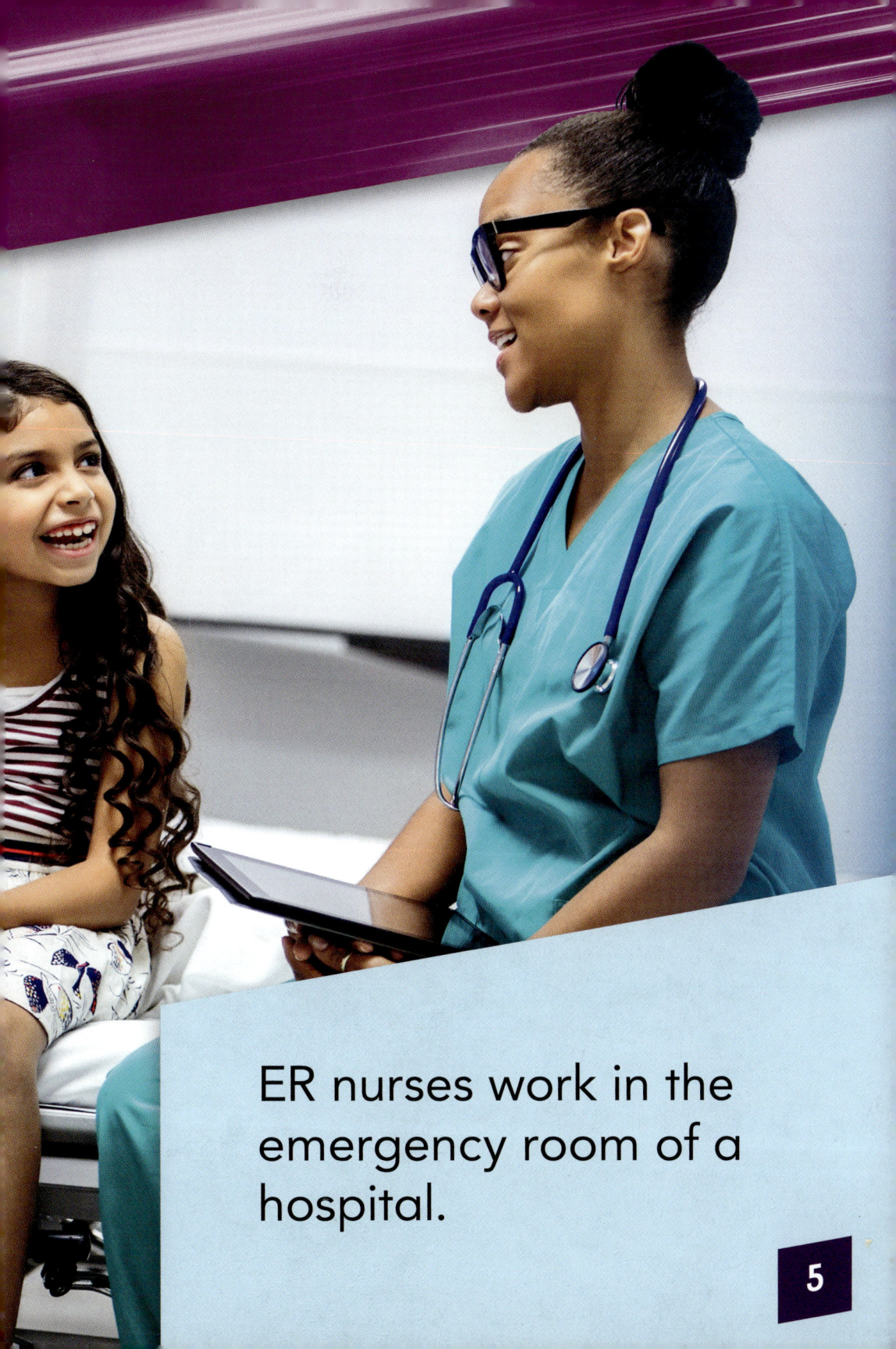

ER nurses work in the emergency room of a hospital.

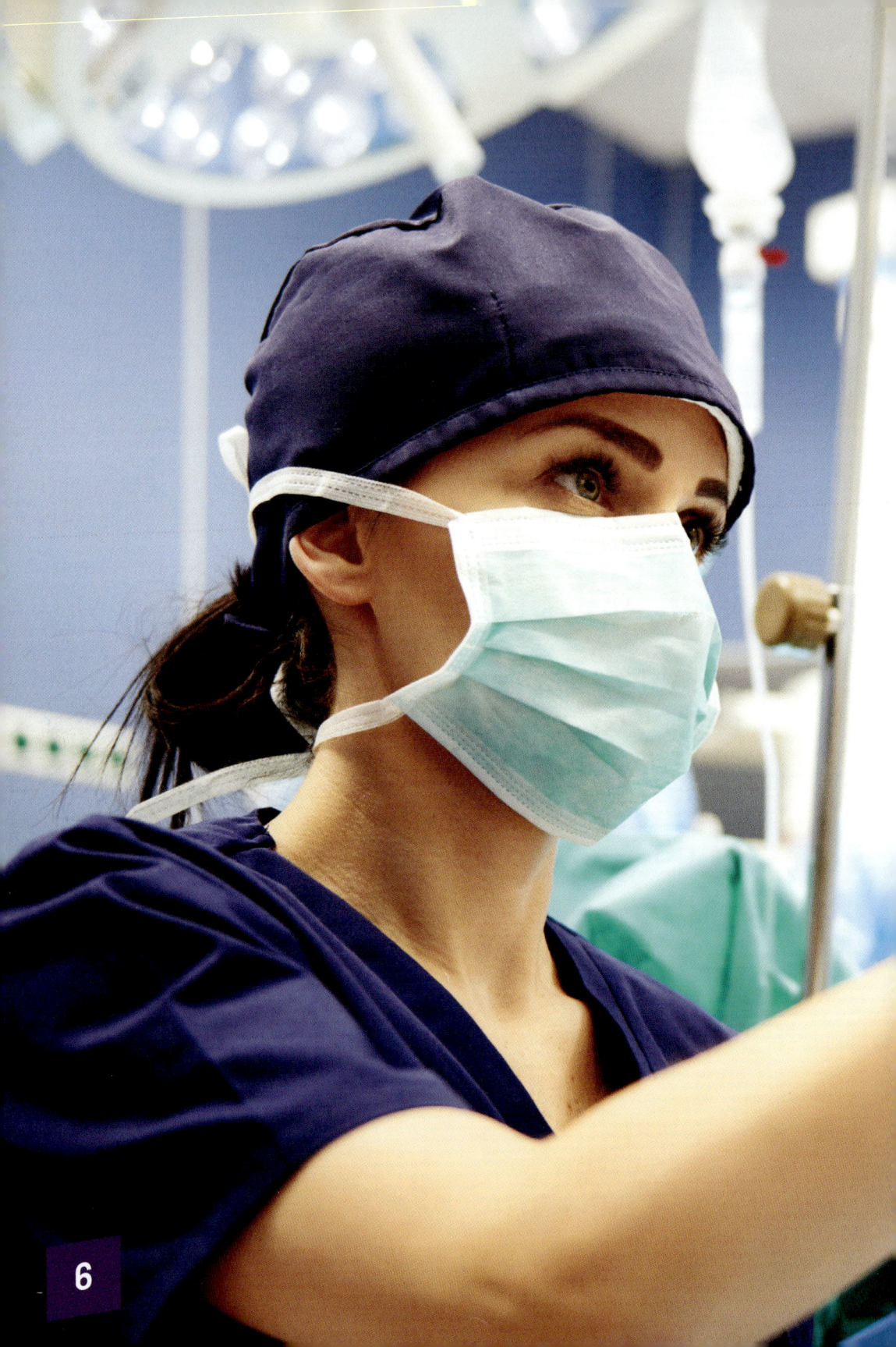

ER nurses have a high-**stress** job. They work at a fast pace!

They treat many serious issues, like heart attacks and broken bones.

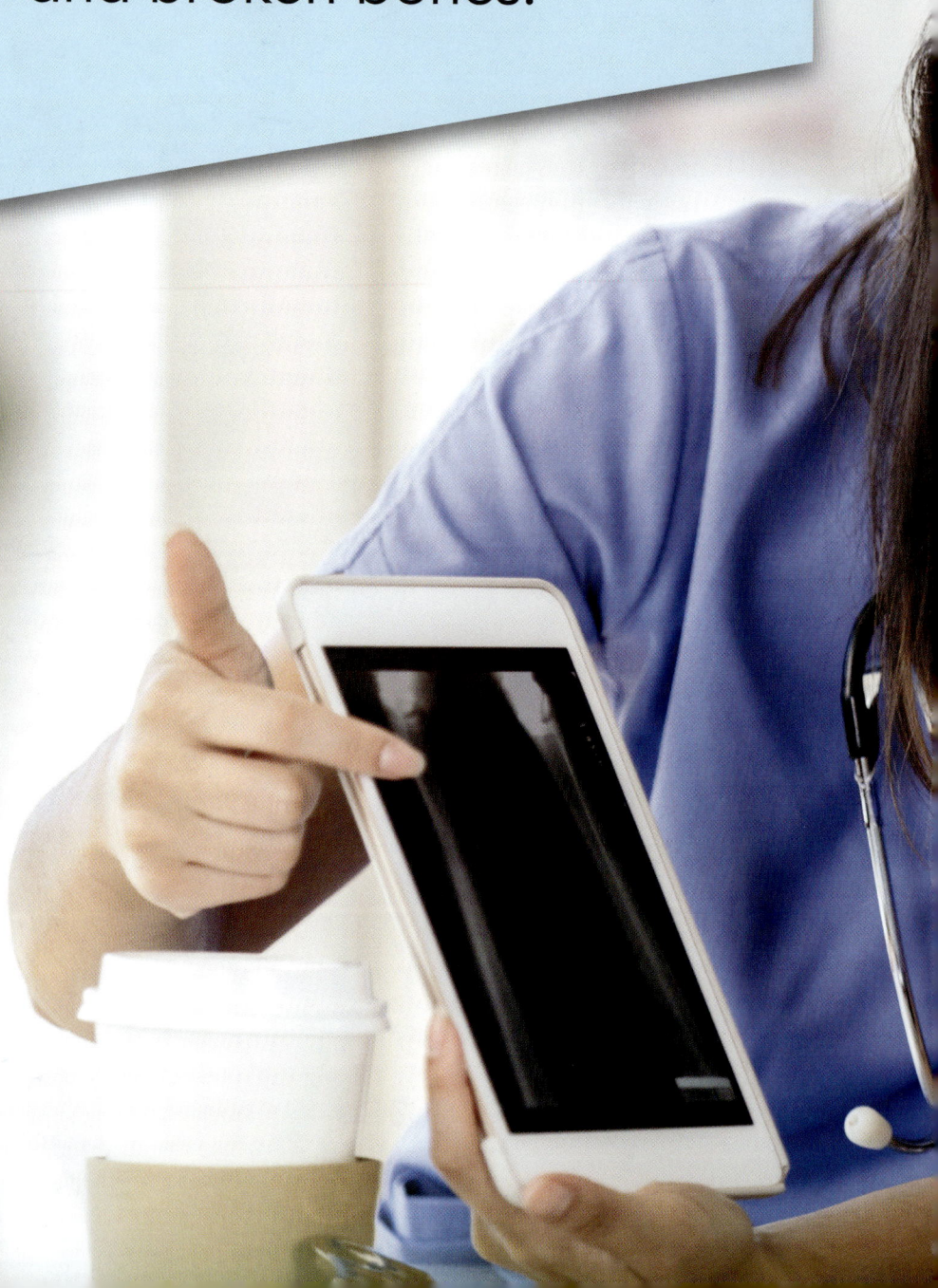

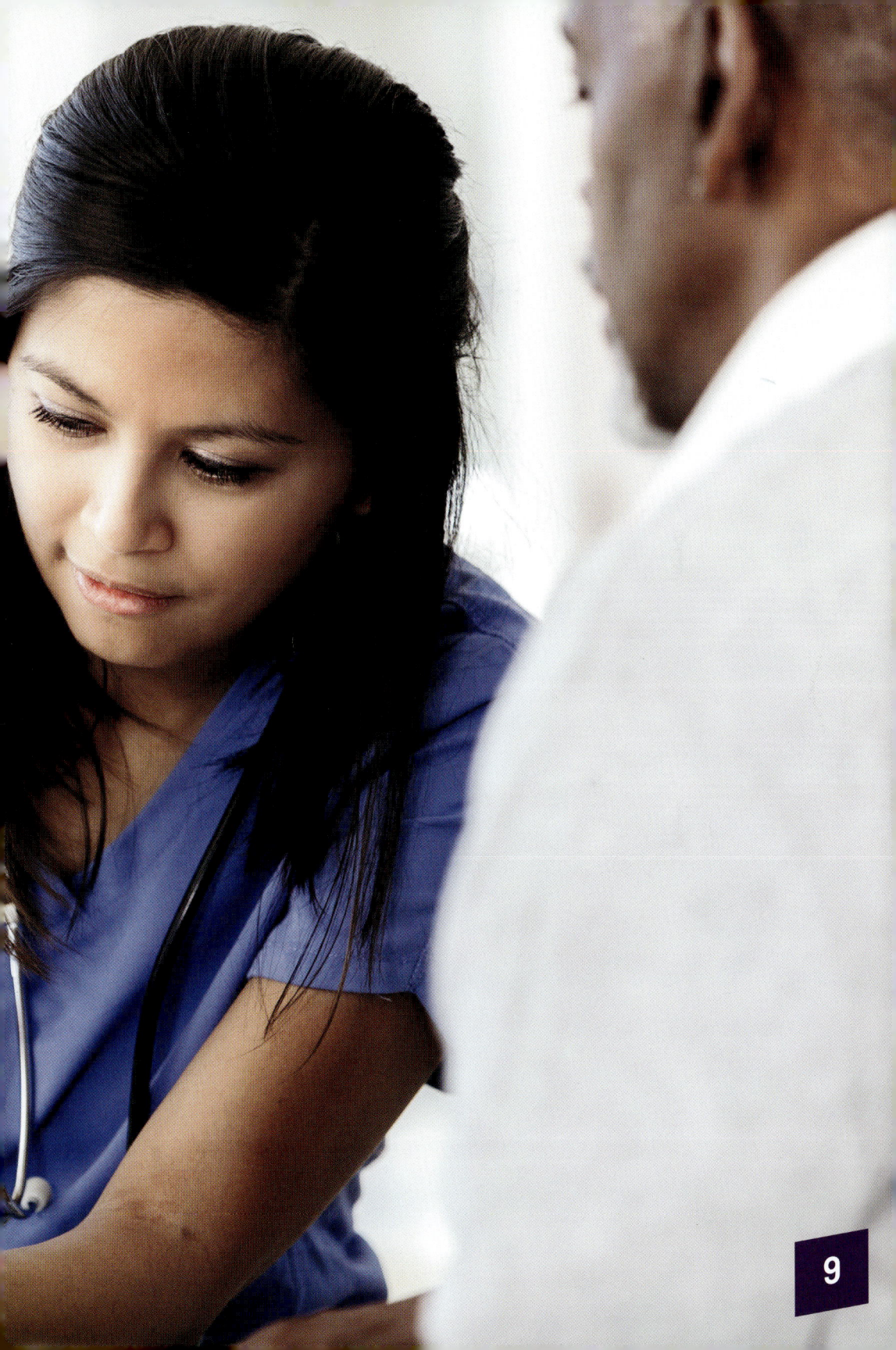

ER nurses quickly **assess** the patient. They make a plan of action.

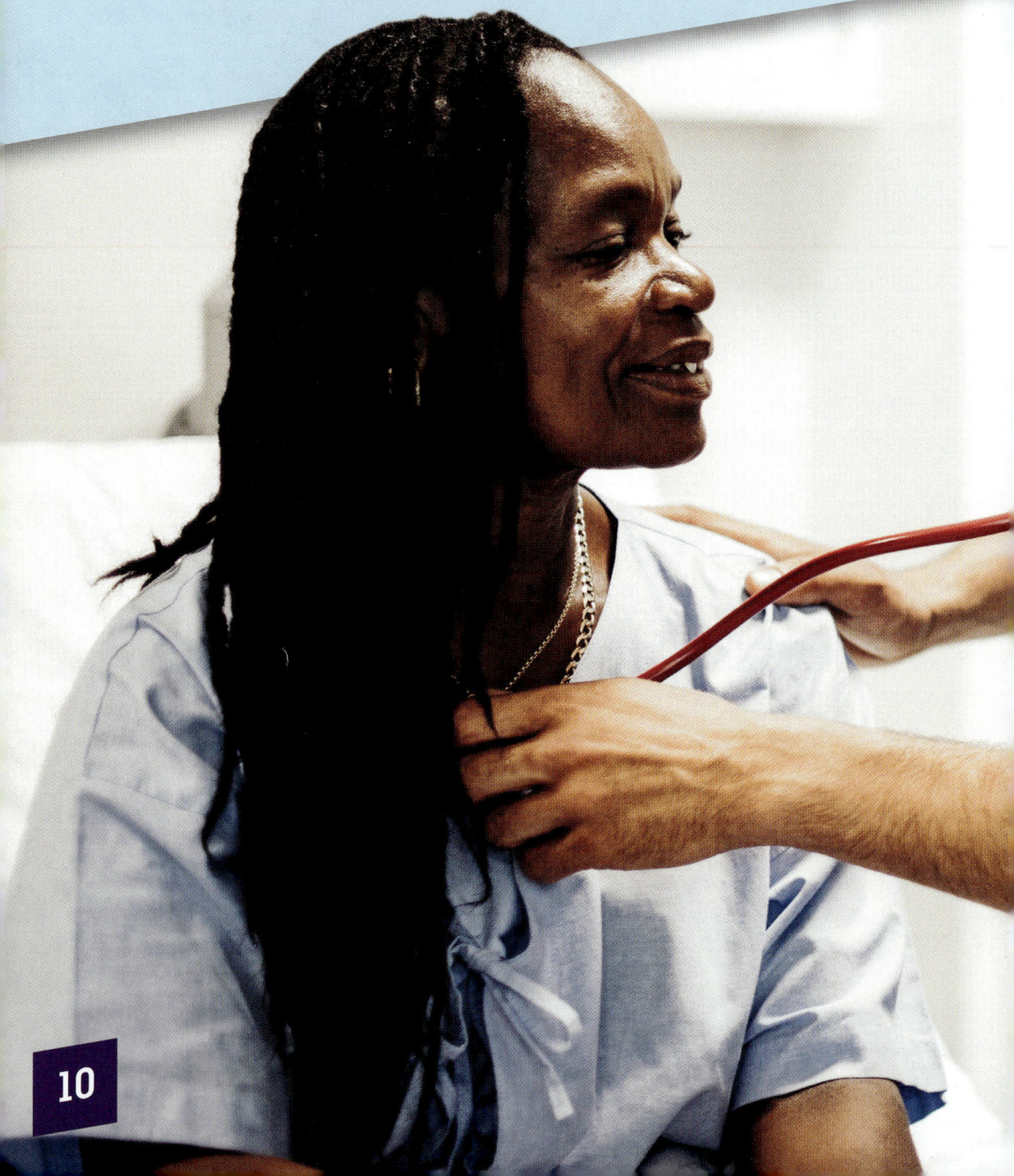

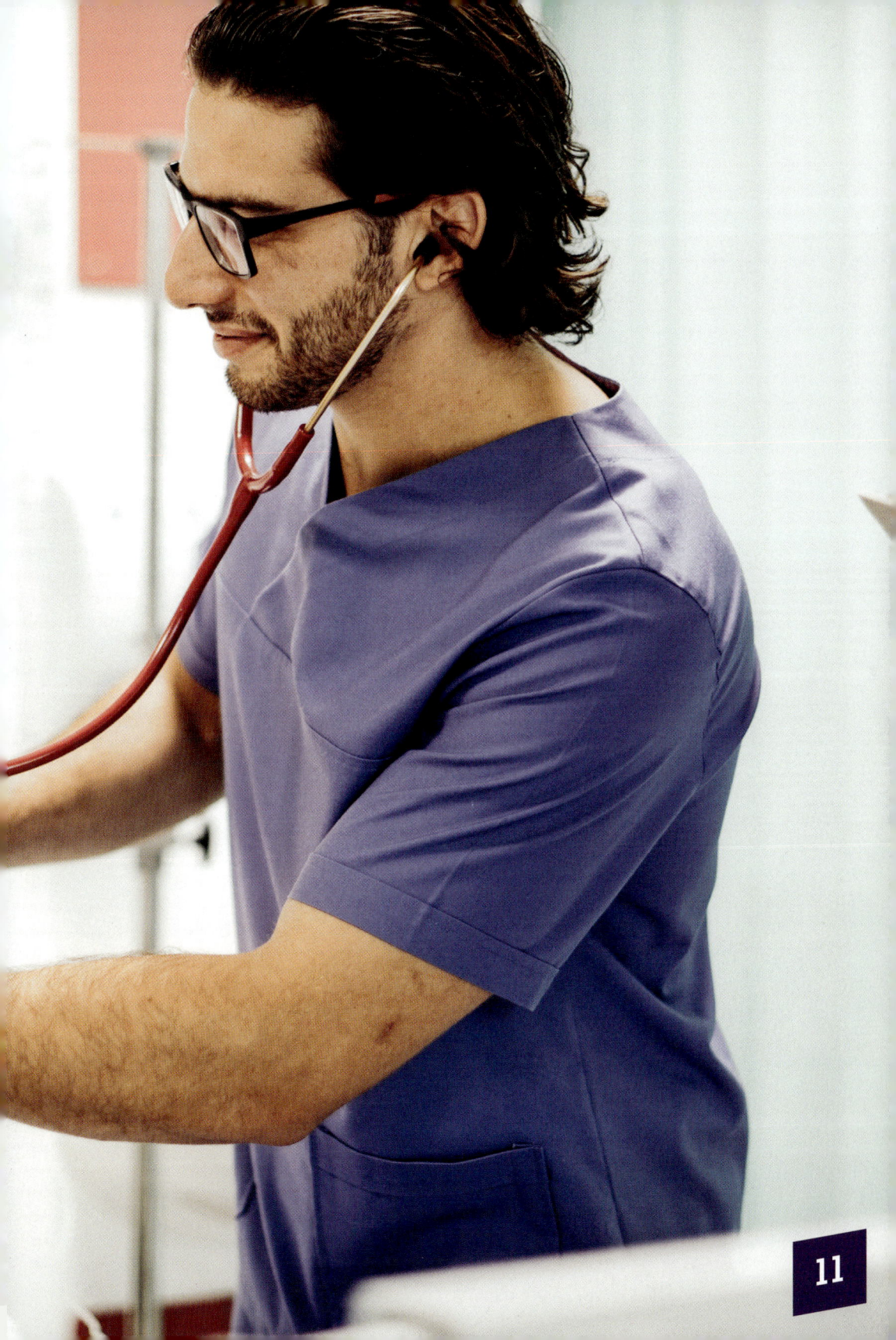

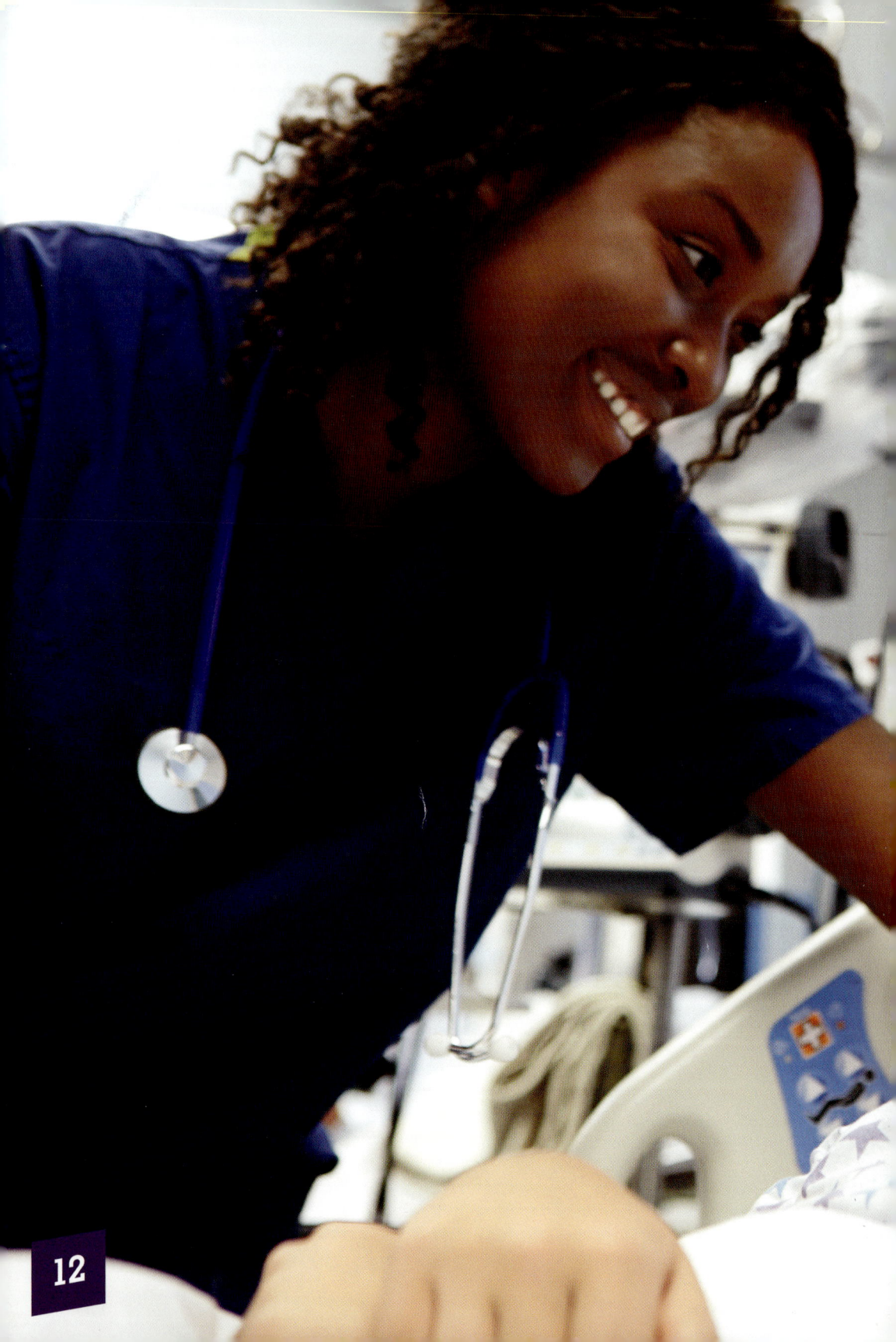

They sometimes have to **stabilize** a patient in failing health. If needed, they can help manage pain.

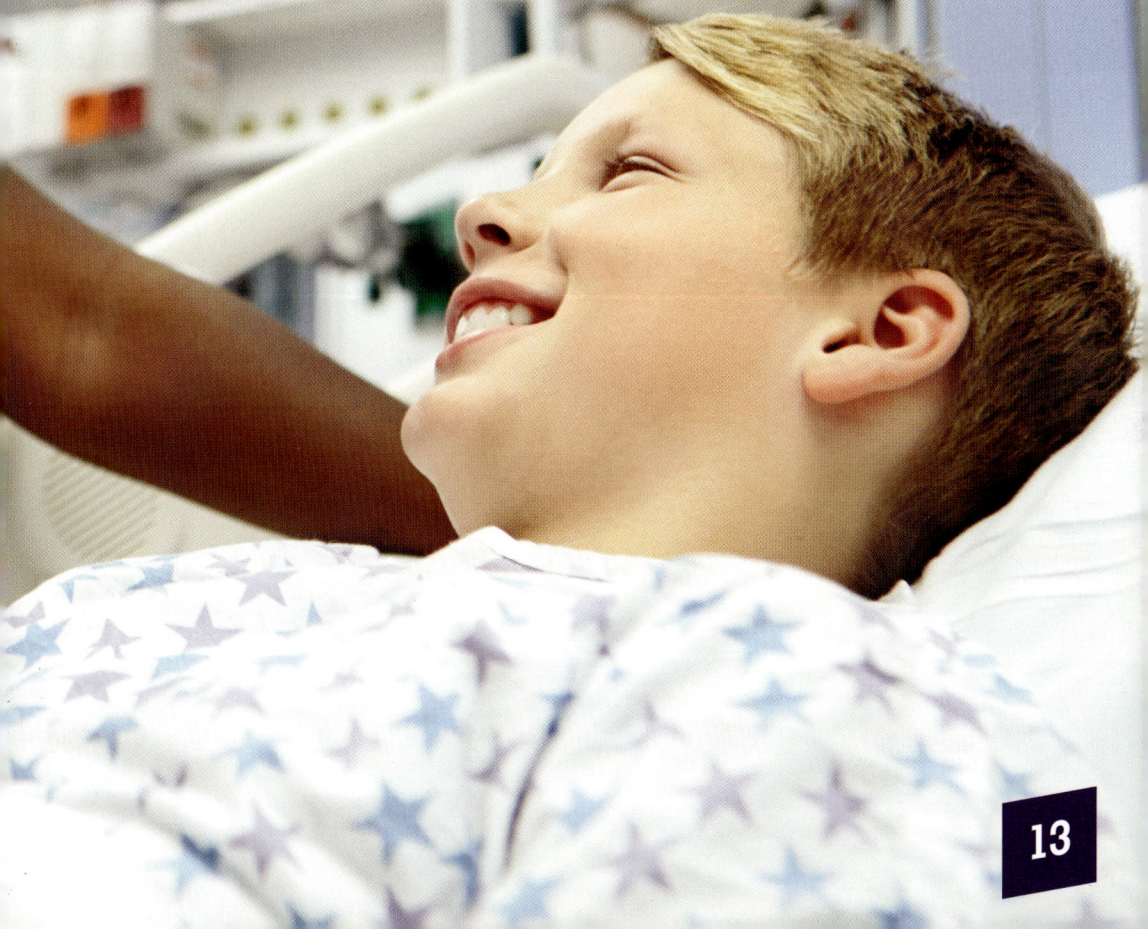

13

ER nurses work closely with ER doctors. They help patients as a team!

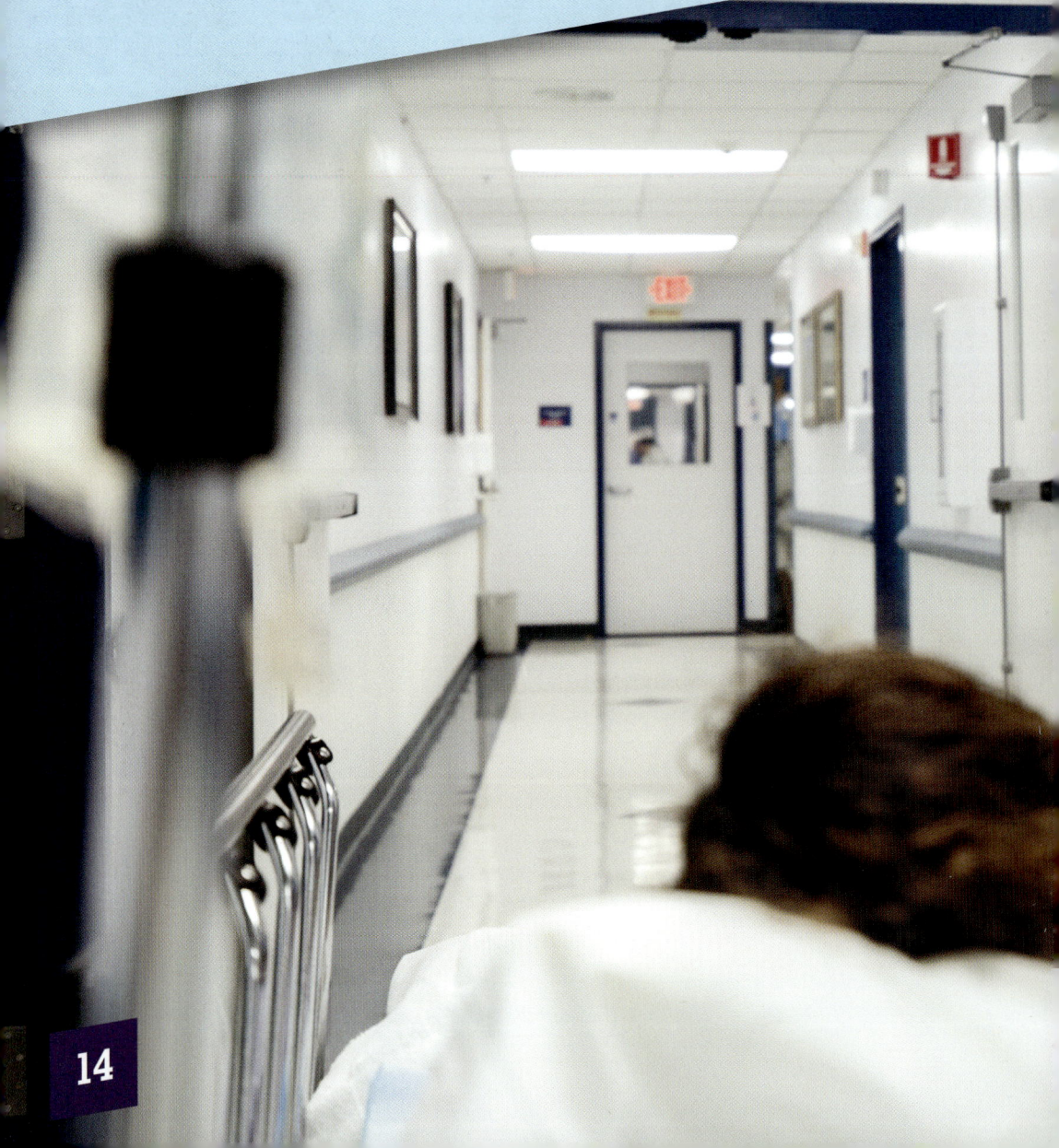

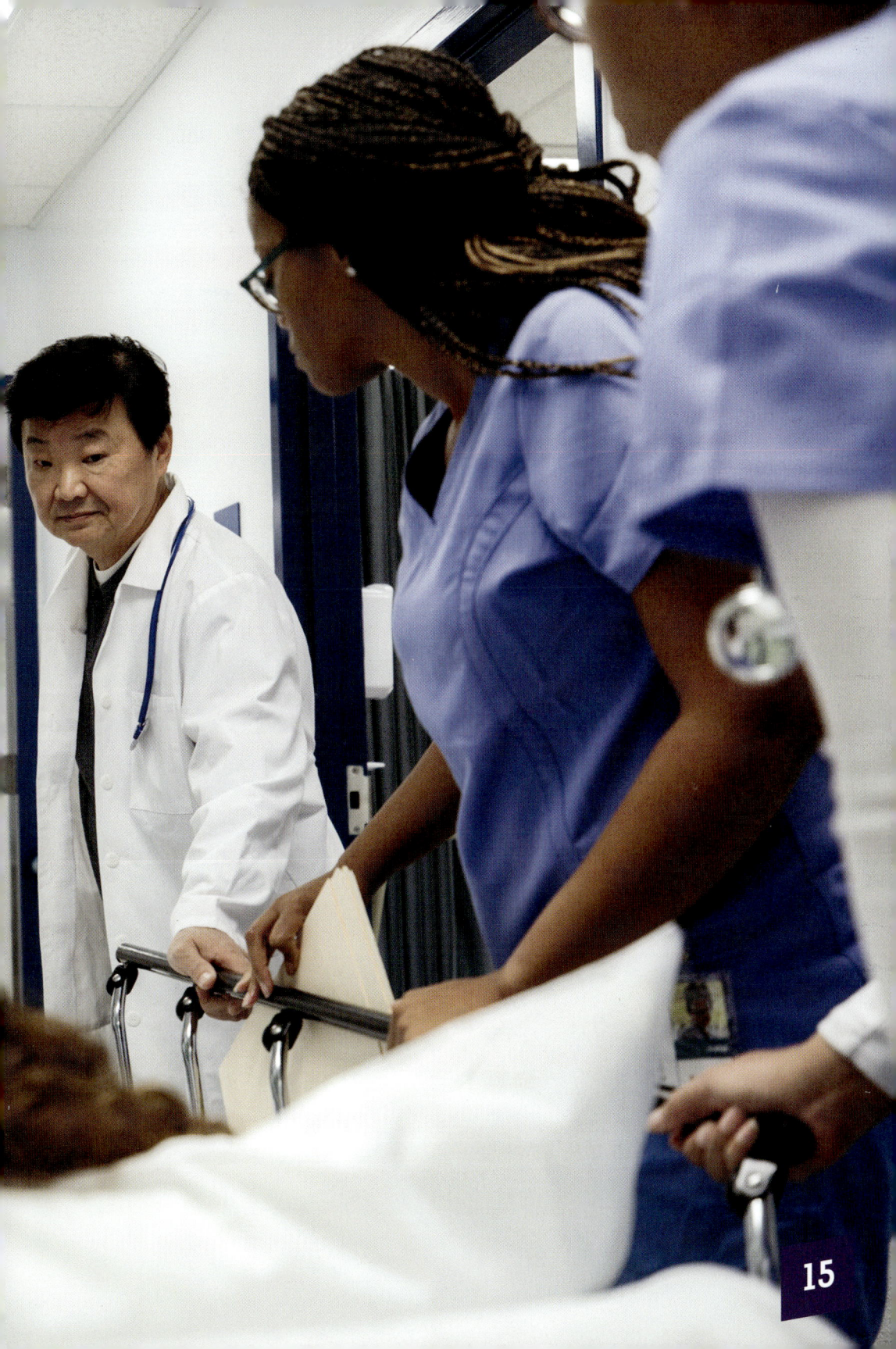

Training

Becoming an ER nurse can take many years. First, one must become a **registered nurse.**

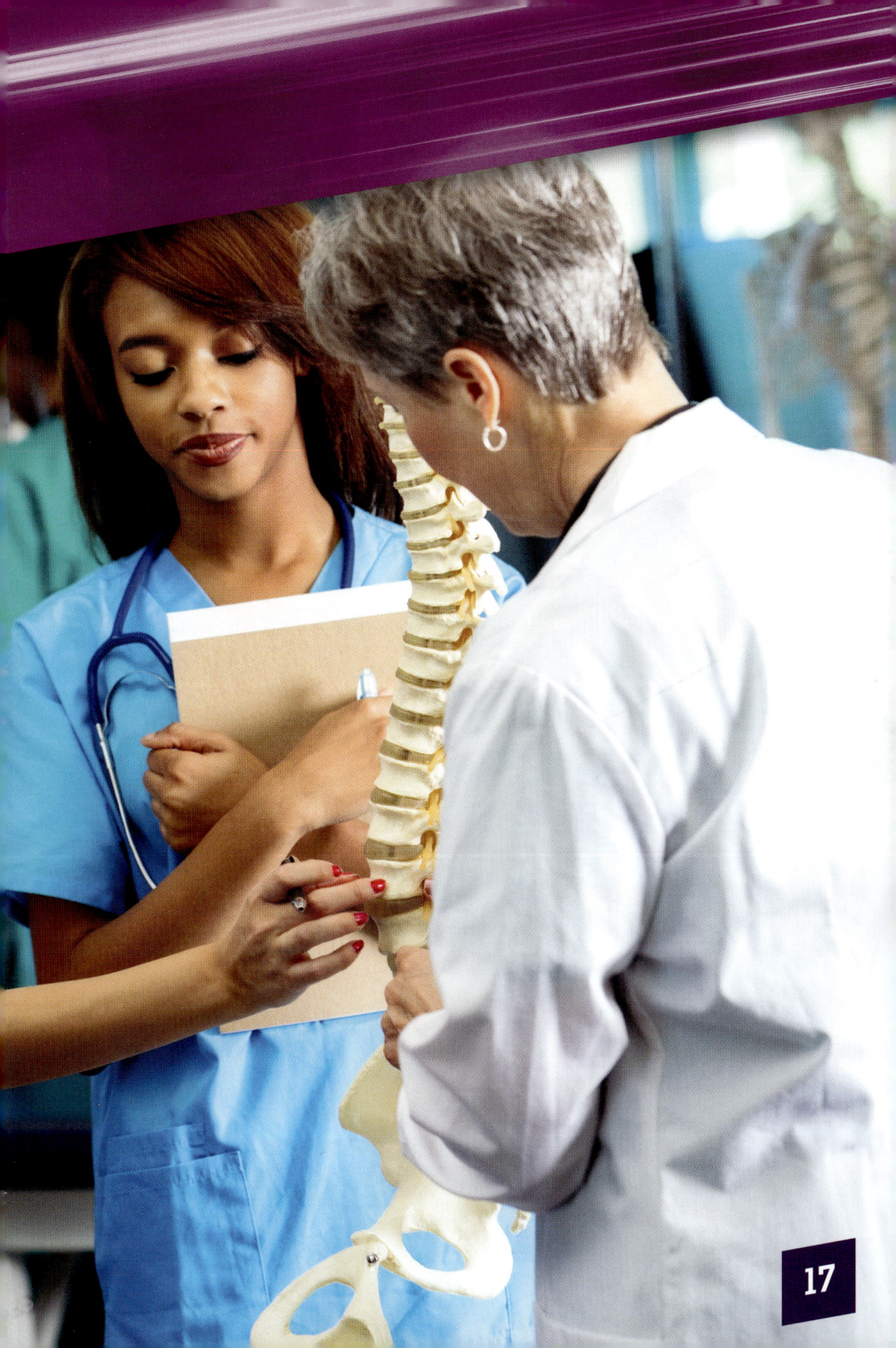

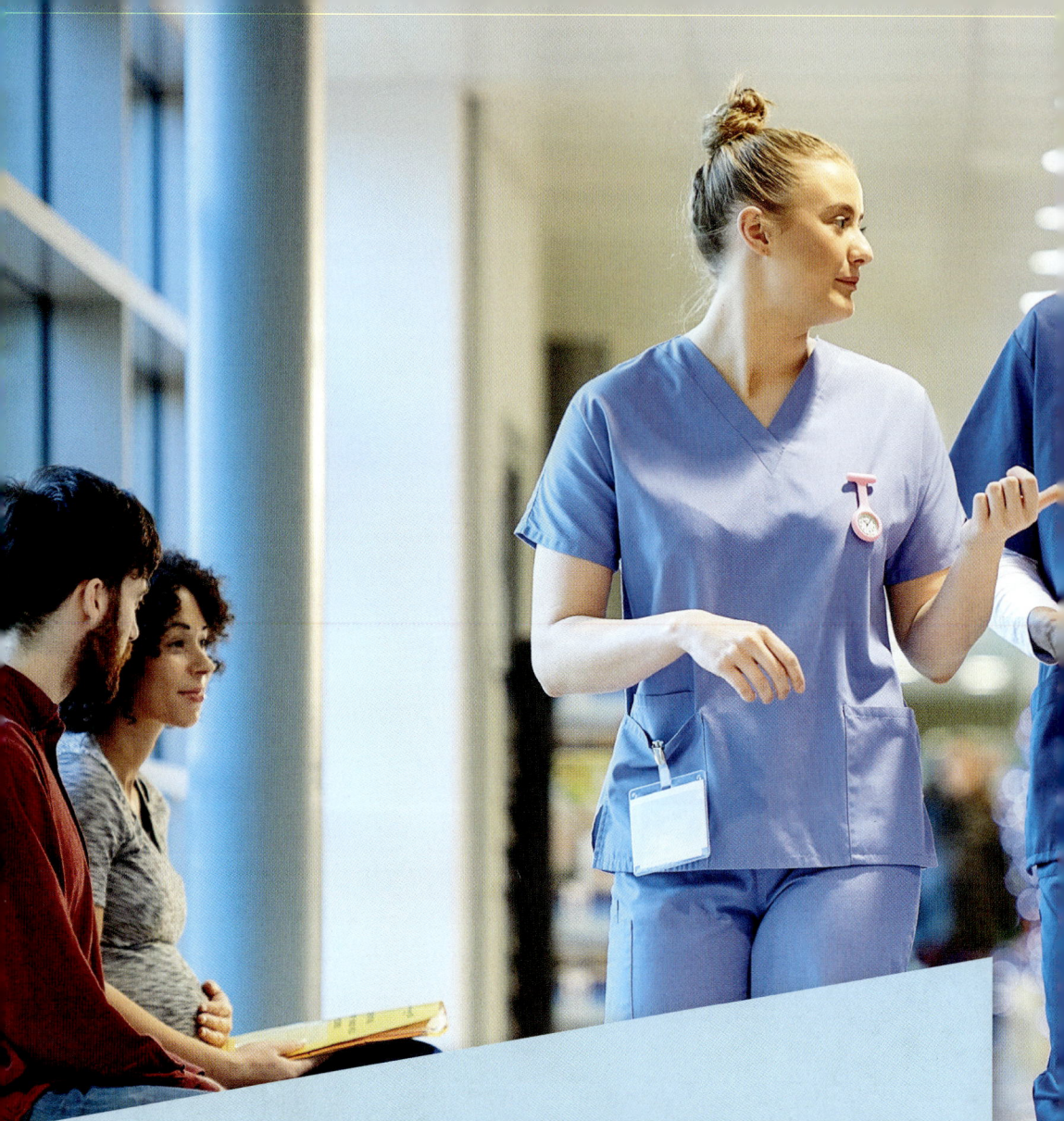

Next, a nurse needs two years of work experience. This must be in emergency medicine.

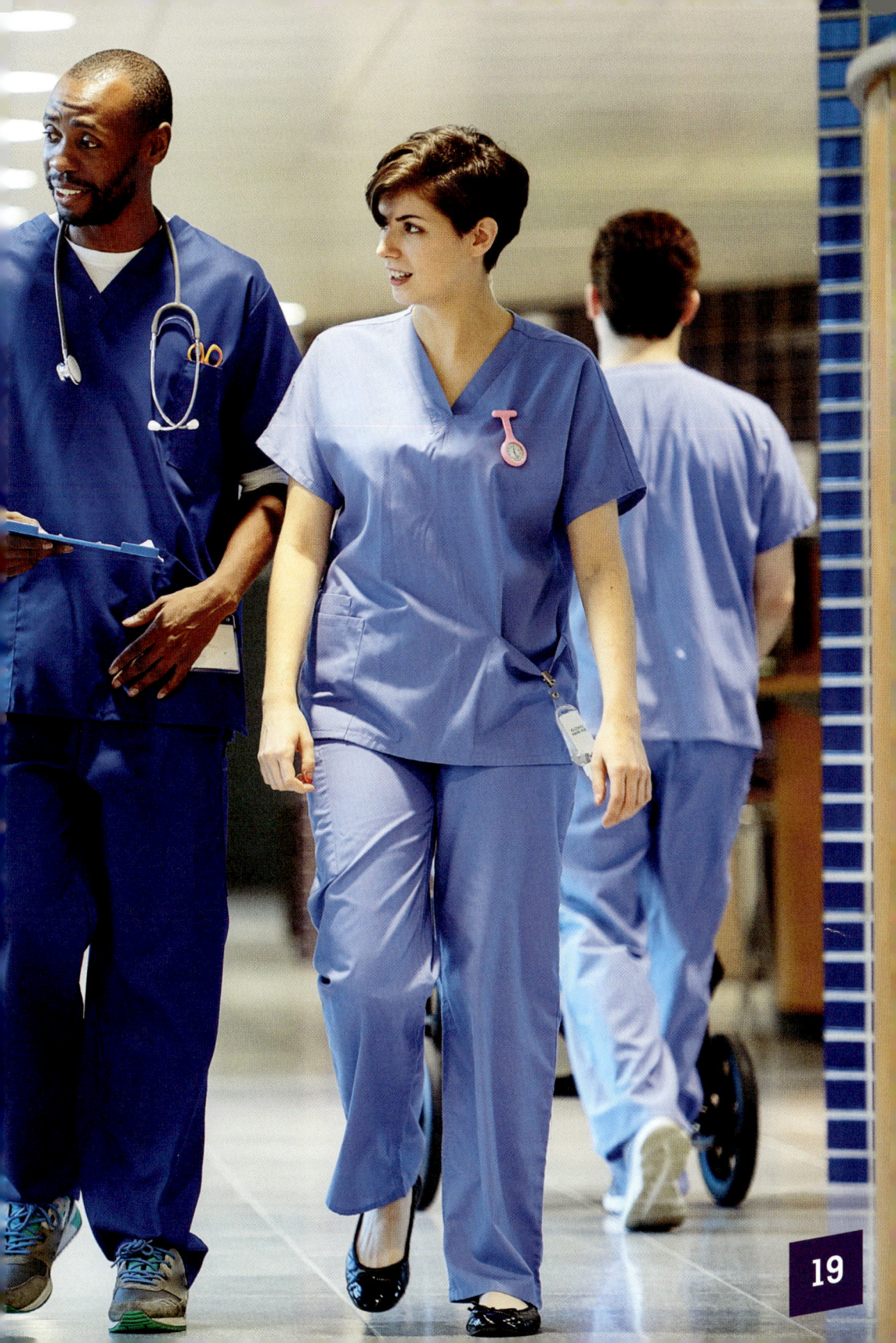

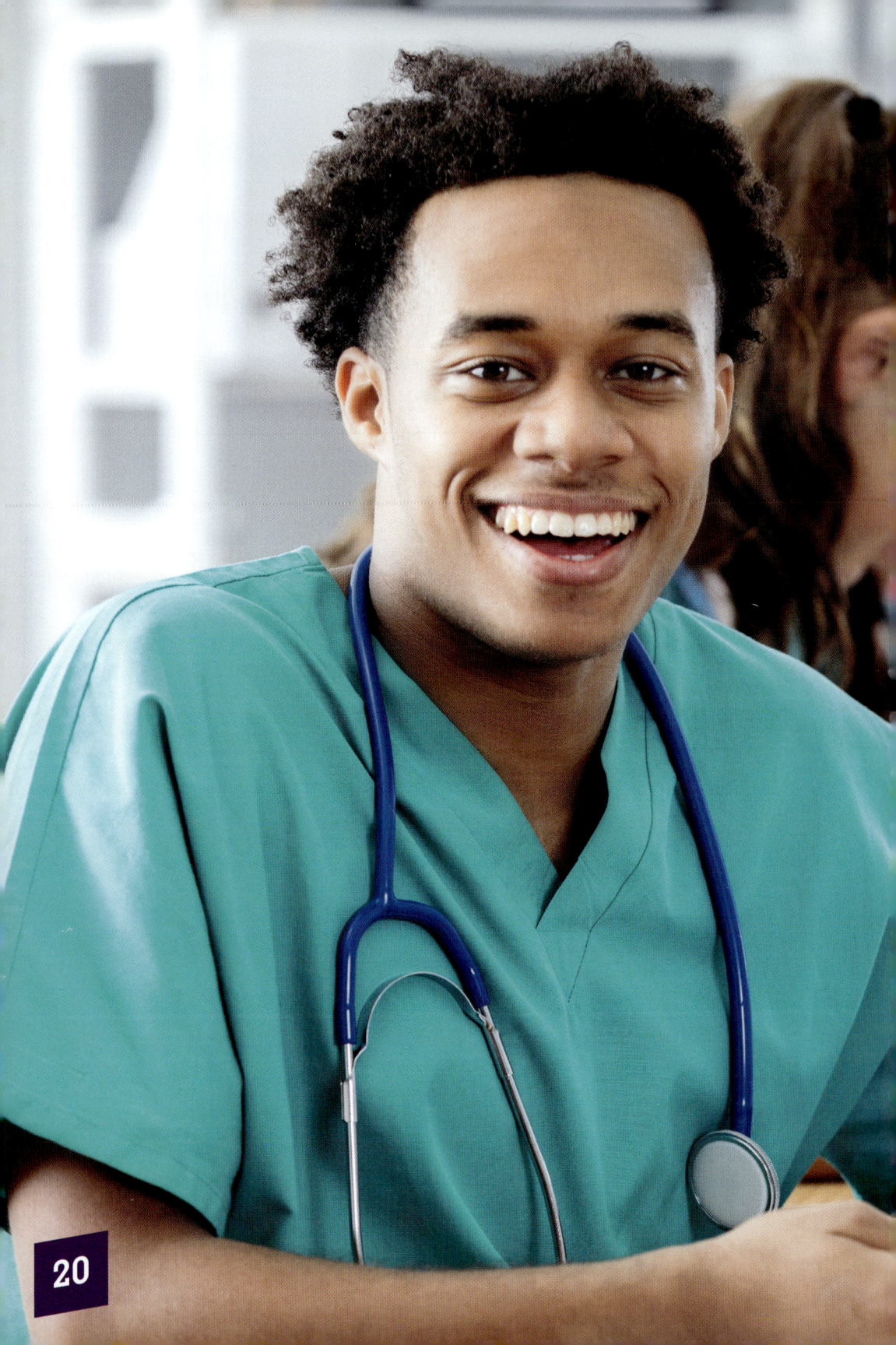

Lastly, a nurse must be **certified** as an ER nurse. This means passing a final exam.

More Facts

- There are about 90,000 emergency nurses in the US.

- National Nurses Day is May 6 in the United States. It kicks off a week of celebrating nurses and ends on May 12, which is Florence Nightingale's birthday.

- Florence Nightingale is the founder of modern nursing.

Glossary

assess – to look at and try to learn the seriousness of something, like an injury.

certified – having earned official certification.

registered nurse – a nurse who has graduated from a college's nursing program or from a school of nursing and has passed a national licensing exam.

stabilize – a process to prevent a critically ill person from having their medical condition decline further.

stress – physical and mental pressure that causes a strain on someone.

Index

Online Resources

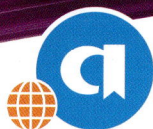

Booklinks
NONFICTION NETWORK
FREE! ONLINE NONFICTION RESOURCES

To learn more about ER nurses, please visit **abdobooklinks.com** or scan this QR code. These links are routinely monitored and updated to provide the most current information available.